MW01679494

# *Your Baby...*

Kevin J. Moore, PhD

Stephanie Moore

FOREWORD BY SHARON MOORE

ISBN: 9798465236638



Edited by Lynell Aycock and Sharon Moore

Cover Design by Estella Vukovic

Printed in the United States

# DEDICATION

We want to express our deepest gratitude to Pregnancy Resource Centers for their faithfulness in empowering women to make life-affirming choices.

# CONTENTS

# FOREWORD

Your Baby…the title of Kevin's book touched my heart because this profound truth is often lost in the fear and upset of an unplanned pregnancy. The voices of parents, boyfriends and a culture that devalues children are loud and persistent. The truth is this…this is your baby. Regardless of the choice of mothers and fathers…this is your baby.

God has a good plan for your child. We could not have imagined God's plan when we held our tiny newborn babies. We did not know how He would use my daughter's little bitty hands to care for the sick with skill and expertise as a physician. We never imagined that our first baby boy would become a missionary and translate the Bible into another language. We did not know that our second son would become a pastor and write this book to give your baby a voice.

Kevin reminds us that your baby is made in God's image and is already loved by God. Your baby has a name and will bring you joy. Your baby needs you right now. As mothers see their babies for the first time on ultrasound, I have seen them look away in anger, then turn their head back to see their baby and cry. This is the moment we know the baby is safe. You are pregnant – don't look away when your baby needs you the most. The Bible says, "Blessed are those who have regard for the weak; the Lord delivers them in times of trouble" (Psalm 41:1). God wants to bless you as you show regard for the baby in your womb! Read this book and love the precious baby that God is giving you. I pray this book will strengthen and encourage you to parent your baby with all your heart.

Sharon Moore
Mother to Three Children
Former Chaplain
Wise Choices Pregnancy Resource Center
Decatur, TX

# MORNING: DAY 1

## *YOUR BABY IS…*

## MADE IN THE IMAGE OF GOD

So God created mankind in his own image,
in the image of God he created them;
male and female he created them.
Genesis 1:27

Have you thought about what your baby might look like? Do you think you are having a boy or a girl? If it's a girl, maybe she will have your eyes. If it's a boy, maybe he will be tall and strong like your dad. There are so many joys to look forward to during your pregnancy journey. Only God knows what your baby will look like. We can be sure of one thing – your baby will be made in the image of God. As you have learned, our world can be so harsh, dark, and cold. Life is filled with hardship and turmoil. In the midst of all the pain and suffering, God is giving you the sweetest reminder of Himself. Your baby is being made in the image of God. What could make your baby more precious and valuable? Your baby is a wonderful gift from God. God shared with your baby aspects of His own nature. When God created the heavens and the earth, He was not content with only the animals of the field and the fish of the sea. The sun, the moon, and the stars are marvelous, but not enough to satisfy God's desire for love and relationship. So, God created humanity in His own image. Your baby shares this desire for love and relationship with God Himself. As you love your baby, even while in the womb, you celebrate the image of God and the wonder of God's creation. Today, spend time giving thanks for the precious reminder of God in your life.

## EVENING PRAYER

Heavenly Father, thank you for creating my baby in your own image. My baby is a precious gift from you. Give me the strength and grace to love my baby. When I am tired and stressed, help me to remember that my baby is the crown of your creation, a living reminder of your image. With every discomfort and trial along the way, help me feel the warmth of your presence as I love and care for the baby that you have placed in my womb. I am trusting you to provide for all my needs as I begin this pregnancy journey. Help me rest well tonight and wake up with fresh energy to do everything that I need to do. In Jesus' name, Amen.

# MORNING: DAY 2

## *Your Baby Is...*

## LOVED BY GOD

For God so loved the world that he gave his one and only Son, that whoever believes in him shall not perish but have eternal life.
John 3:16

God loves your baby! In fact, you can't even believe how much God loves your baby. God knew that your child would one day sin and need a Savior. So, God made a way for your child to one day be forgiven. God sent His Son Jesus to live the perfect life. Since Jesus lived the perfect life, He served as the perfect sacrifice for the sins of the world. Jesus died on the cross so that those who believe can have eternal life.

It might seem hard to love a baby that you

have never met, but not for God. God's love for your child is massive! Since God loves your baby, one of the greatest acts of obedience is to bring this beautiful child into the world. God will reward you for this obedience.

Did you know that God loves you too? God loves you more than you could ever imagine. He knows all about the things that you have done and said. He knows about every bad decision you have ever made, but He still loves you. God loves you just as much as He loves your baby.

Have you ever trusted Jesus Christ to forgive you of your sins? God loved you so much that He sent his precious Son Jesus to the earth. Unlike all of us, Jesus lived the perfect life and died for us. On the third day, God raised Jesus to new life. As we express faith in the Lord Jesus as the Son of God and turn from our sin – we can be completely forgiven. The resurrection of Jesus from the grave gives us the wonderful privilege of living a new life that is pleasing to God.

God loves you and He wants you to love Him back. He wants you to spend eternity in a perfect place called Heaven. If you have never become a Christian, now is the perfect time to place your faith and trust in Jesus Christ for the forgiveness of your sins. Right now, you can bow your head, express faith in Jesus and ask Him to save you from your sins. Right now, you can ask the Lord to make you His daughter!

## EVENING PRAYER

Heavenly Father, I know that I am a sinner. I believe that you loved me so much that you sent your Son Jesus to die for my sin on the cross. Jesus – I believe that you are the Savior. God, I believe that you raised Jesus from the dead on the third day. I want to follow you and obey you the rest of my life. Forgive me for all the sin in my life. Help me to turn from these sins and live my life for you. I want to read the Bible and pray so that I can know you more. Thank you for loving me and thank you for saving me. Let me become your daughter. In Jesus' name, Amen.

# MORNING: DAY 3

## *YOUR BABY IS...*

## CREATED TO DO GREAT THINGS

For we are God's handiwork, created in Christ Jesus to do good works, which God prepared in advance for us to do.
Ephesians 2:10

This very minute, God is uniquely creating your child to do great things. God has a very special purpose for your child! Maybe your child will become a famous musician that will amaze the world with beautiful melodies. Or maybe your child will develop the first cure for some terminal disease. Maybe your baby will become a pastor who will spend his life preaching the Bible. Maybe your child will become a powerful politician or an inspirational teacher. Whatever the plan is, it is going to be great! You are on a wonderful journey to see just how incredible God's plan is for your child.

Speaking of "good works," as a mother you already are doing one of the good works that God has prepared you to do. You are doing a good work by creating a safe, loving environment for your baby to grow and develop. In fact, raising your child just may be the most important thing that you will ever do with your life. May the Lord bless you as you continue this good work!

## EVENING PRAYER

Heavenly Father, thank you for calling me to this good work of motherhood. Thank you for giving me all the grace and the strength that I need to persevere through this exciting journey that I am on. Some days I feel like I do not have the strength to be a good mother. Give me everything that I need to be the mother that you have called me to be. Prepare in advance a great work for my child. Help my baby to accomplish things that have never been done. Let my child bring beauty, creativity, and joy into the world. Help me to recognize giftedness and shepherd my child toward the great work that you have already prepared. In Jesus' name, Amen.

## MORNING: DAY 4

*YOUR BABY IS...*

# KNIT TOGETHER BY GOD

For you created my inmost being;
you knit me together in my mother's womb. I will give thanks to You, because I am awesomely and wonderfully made; Wonderful are Your works, and my soul knows it very well.
Psalm 139:13-14

Leonardo da Vinci's *Salvator Mundi* sold in 2016 to Saudi Arabia's Crown prince for more than 450 million dollars, making it the most expensive artwork ever sold at auction. It is difficult to fathom having that kind of money. Did you know that your baby is worth much more? In fact, your baby is priceless. Your baby's Creator is infinitely more creative than Leonardo da Vinci. Even now, God is knitting your baby together in your womb.

God knows the kind of person your baby will become. God knows exactly what your baby is going to do when he or she grows up. In fact, God knows every detail about their future. With God's comprehensive knowledge, He knows exactly how to make your child. Even now, God is knitting your baby together in the most wonderful way possible.

Every detail about your baby represents the ingenious design of Almighty God, from the color of eyes and hair to the baby's skin tone and facial features. God is even crafting the inmost being of your baby. In ways that we cannot even begin to understand, God is perfectly crafting your child into who He who wants your child to become. God does not make mistakes. Your baby will be awesome in every way.

Can you even imagine how glorious it is going to be to meet your baby for the very first time? It won't be long. Today, spend time giving thanks to God for this priceless gift. Thank God for making your child perfect in every way. Ask God for the strength and endurance to wait while He fearfully and wonderfully knits your child together.

## EVENING PRAYER

Heavenly Father, even though I cannot see my baby, your eyes can. My baby is being handcrafted by you in amazing ways; unique and beautiful, like no other person on this earth. Right now, these tiny fingers already have their very own fingerprint. I pray that my child will use these hands that you have made to do great things. I look forward to the day that these tiny fingers will wrap around mine and we will hold hands for the first time. Nourish my body so that my baby can grow bigger and stronger every day. Nourish my heart and my soul so that I can help my baby grow into the person you want them to be. In Jesus' name, Amen.

# MORNING: DAY 5

## *YOUR BABY...*

## HAS A NAME

Listen to me, you islands;
hear this, you distant nations:
Before I was born the LORD called me;
from my mother's womb
he has spoken my name.
Isaiah 49:1

Did you know that your baby already has a name? Even before you settle on a name, God already knows your baby's name. Your baby is not fetal tissue to Almighty God. Your baby is a person, and every person has a name. Even before your baby is born God is speaking their name. Isn't that wonderful?

I don't think that God will ever stop calling your child's name. For the rest of his or her life, God will call out to your child. God will call your child to faith, obedience, holiness, worship, and service. God will call to your child when they are about to make a bad decision. He will call their name when they need strength to do the right thing. He will call their name at times, just to tell your child that He loves them. Throughout every high and low in life, God will shepherd your child by calling their name.

Have you thought about what to name your baby? It's not too early to start thinking about it. Is there a special person in your life whose name you would love to give to your baby? Maybe you want to name the baby after a beloved family member. Is there a name that you have always loved? After you decide on a name, you can join God in calling to your baby using their name. Talk to your baby. Sing to your baby. Pray for your baby using their name. Let your child get used to hearing you speak their name even while they are in the womb. If you don't have a name yet, don't panic, you still have time. Spend a few moments asking God what He wants you to name your child.

## EVENING PRAYER

Heavenly Father, You already know my baby and know my baby's name. Even now, you might be whispering your love to my baby by name. What an incredible thought this is to me. With billions of people in the world, you still want to know my baby by name. As my child grows, I pray that my baby would love you back and call your name. I'm also thankful that you know my name. You have not once forgotten me during this challenging time in my life. Thank you for your love for me and for wanting to be the most important part of my life. Help me to call upon your name for help when I need it. In Jesus' name, Amen.

## MORNING: DAY 6

*YOUR BABY...*

## WILL GIVE YOU JOY

A woman giving birth to a child has pain because her time has come; but when her baby is born she forgets the anguish because of her joy that a child is born into the world.
John 16:21

We have all seen that dramatic moment of childbearing in the movies. You can expect to see a young man rushing his pregnant wife to the hospital, dodging cars, and careening dangerously through rush-hour traffic. In Hollywood fashion, there is plenty of drama with the birthing experience as well. There might be a dad passing out, a police officer pulling over the speeding father, or possibly even a fireman delivering the baby on the side of the busy interstate. Of course, all of this is accompanied by the deafening screams of a woman who arrived too late to enjoy the anesthesiologic bliss of an epidural. I think we can all agree Hollywood goes way over the top. Let's face it, though, delivering a baby can be painful. Did you know that there is something far more intense than the physical pain of childbirth?

Joy. John 16:21 says it is so well, "but when her baby is born she forgets the anguish because of her joy..." Even if the Hollywood version of having a baby was completely accurate, it can't possibly capture the joy that a mother feels in her heart when she holds her baby for the very first time. The discomfort of having a baby is no match for this joy. This joy will be better than any other joy you have experienced. This joy will make every other happy moment in your life seem so very small. This joy is more overwhelming than the pain of giving birth. In fact, the Bible says that it is so powerful that the mother "forgets the anguish." Are you ready for this kind of joy? It will not be long. Hang in there and keep up the good work.

With every discomfort, I want you to think about the joy that is coming your way. Every time you are nauseous, achy, or fatigued, remember the joy that God promised. Let every physically uncomfortable moment prompt you to look forward to the unspeakable joy that's on its way. You can do this!

## EVENING PRAYER

Heavenly Father, I feel scared to deliver this baby. I don't know what to expect. The Bible tells me I will experience joy – so I'm trusting you. As I continue to carry this baby inside my womb, give me the energy and health I need. It is hard to imagine seeing my baby for the first time, but I am so excited. One day, this baby will be placed in my arms and I will gaze into the eyes of this beautiful baby I have prayed for. Help me to endure the hardship of each day, knowing that I have something wonderful to look forward to. Help me to get a great night of sleep tonight and awake rested in the morning. In Jesus' name, Amen.

# MORNING: DAY 7

## *YOUR BABY...*

## NEEDS YOU

Yet you brought me out of the womb;
you made me trust in you,
even at my mother's breast.
Psalm 22:9

Being young and carefree is one of the greatest joys in life. Getting to spend your afternoons however you want. Going wherever you want, whenever you want. Life never stays this way, though. As we grow up, God allows us the privilege of having more responsibility. It's not a bad thing; it's a natural part of maturing into the person God wants you to be. Now that you are pregnant, you need to start thinking less about yourself and more about your baby.

Your baby desperately needs you right now. Nobody can provide for your baby like you can. You are uniquely situated to provide for your baby.

Nobody else can protect your baby the way that you can right now. Nobody else can make sure that your baby receives the nutrients needed to grow properly while in the womb. Nobody else can take prenatal vitamins and eat healthy to help your child develop. God wants you to do it. God chose you to do it. There may be plenty of people in your life that need you in their life right now, but your baby needs you more than anybody. Most of the people who put pressure on you are capable of doing things for themselves. Your baby, however, is counting on you. He or she cannot do anything on their own.

Make your child a priority today. Get the rest that you need every night. Make healthy choices so that your baby can grow strong. Say "no" to anything and everything that might hurt you or your child. Ask the Lord for strength to quit any bad habits that are harmful. Stay away from bad influences and only spend time with people who truly care about you.

Don't let your new responsibilities frighten you. Few things in life are more rewarding than being the one person that your child depends on more than anybody else in the world. It is a joy and a privilege to care for your baby. As you care for your child, God will bless you beyond anything you thought possible.

## EVENING PRAYER

Heavenly Father, I am overwhelmed that my baby will be completely dependent upon me. This is a new thought for me. I know I can't do this without you. I do not want to let my baby down. Help me to let go of bad habits and have the strength to say "no" to things that could hurt my child. Please help me stay away from people that don't value my child. Help me to be the mother that my baby needs to grow into a healthy person. Help me to make my baby feel loved and cared for. Give me the determination to make good choices. In Jesus' name, Amen.

# MORNING: DAY 8

## *YOUR BABY...*

## WANTS YOUR COMFORT

As a mother comforts her child, so will I comfort you; and you will be comforted over Jerusalem.
Isaiah 66:13

The Bible teaches that God is the "Father of compassion and the God of all comfort" (2 Cor 1:3). Our God is perfect in His power to comfort His people. How can God get us to understand just how wonderful His comfort is? God uses the picture of a mother comforting her child. This is the most wonderful example of comfort.

God has given you the very special gift of being able to comfort your child. Nobody can comfort like a mother. Friends and coworkers may try to console, but nothing feels like the comfort of a mother. Not even fathers can comfort in the same way that a mother can. God uses that strong connection that you have with your baby to send His love and compassion through you.

Did you know that your baby needs comfort? There will be so many things that your baby does not understand. Your baby will be frightened and lonely at times. In discomfort and pain your baby will reach for you. Sometimes, without any reason at all, your baby will want your comfort.

Mothers also need comfort. Where do moms go when they need comfort? You may have a mother to turn to for comfort or you may not. Either way, God is willing to comfort you "as a mother comforts her child." Run to the Lord when you are tired and frustrated. Seek the Lord when you are burdened and confused. God promises to comfort you. Take a moment to tell the Lord about all the things that are troubling you right now. Ask the Lord to comfort you in the midst of your circumstances. You are not alone in this pregnancy journey!

## EVENING PRAYER

Heavenly Father, I am scared. This is one of the most challenging times of my life. I don't know where the money is going to come from. I know nothing about being a mother. My body aches. People around me don't understand what I am going through. I don't know who to turn to. If you are the God of all comfort, please comfort me right now. Help me sense the warmth of your presence. I am thankful that I am not alone. You are with me. Help me to provide this same sense of warmth and comfort to my baby. Help me to make my baby feel safe and loved. I need you to help me be a good mother. In Jesus' name, Amen.

# MORNING: DAY 9

*Your Baby...*

## WILL BRING YOU HAPPINESS

He settles the childless woman in her home as a happy mother of children. Praise the LORD.
Psalm 113:9

Right now there are countless thousands of women who would love to be in your shoes. Many have prayed and longed for years but have not been able to conceive. Their hearts ache every time they hear a baby cry. Being pregnant can be difficult when you don't know how you are going to raise a child. But consider for a moment just how blessed you are.

Psalm 113:9 describes the mother of children as happy. It might be hard to imagine right now, but you are going to go home from the hospital in a few months as a happy mother. You will be exhausted and ready to sleep all the way through the night, but still happy. One day you will look back over your life and wonder what you ever did to deserve such a wonderful blessing. Your baby is not a disruption or inconvenience in your life. Your baby is a wonderful blessing from God that will bring you more happiness than you can even imagine.

Sometimes when we are tired and stressed, it helps to find something to look forward to. Today, take a moment to think about the happiest memories that you had growing up as a child. Maybe you enjoyed these moments with your mother or maybe your grandfather. Think about all the happy experiences that you want to have with your children. Dream about your baby's first birthday party. Think about taking your son or daughter out for their first snow cone or ice cream. What's your favorite song or music group that you want to introduce your baby to when they get old enough? Every time you get worried or concerned, go back to all these experiences that you look forward to having with your baby.

## EVENING PRAYER

Heavenly Father, every time I start to worry, help me to focus on the happy memories I will make with my child. When I'm stressed and tired, keep me focused on all the wonderful things that I have to look forward to. Someday this baby is going to grow up and want to give me hugs and goodnight kisses. Thank you that I get to be there when my baby learns to crawl and talk. I pray that, when my child grows up, we will have the joy of being best friends. Help me to sleep with peace tonight, knowing that I have so much to look forward to. In Jesus' name, Amen.

# MORNING: DAY 10

*YOUR BABY...*

## HAS HAIR

And even the very hairs of your head
are all numbered.
Matthew 10:30

Did you know that your baby's hair follicles start to form around the 14th week of pregnancy? Wow – that's incredible! Your baby probably has hair already. This hair will grow, then fall off and regrow in cycles during your pregnancy. It will be so exciting to see how much hair your baby has when you deliver!

God knows everything about your baby, including the number of hairs. God created the heavens and the earth, but He still wants to know everything that there is to know about your baby. God took the time to count the hairs on your baby's head. Your baby is more important to God than you could ever imagine.

Since your baby is important to God, take time today to do at least one thing to get ready for the delivery. Have you chosen a doctor to deliver the baby yet? Or, you could pick out an infant car seat so that you can bring your baby home from the hospital after delivery. If you've already done those things, you could shop for a baby bag to hold the diapers, formula, baby powder, and other baby gear. You are also going to need a crib. Some of these things can get pricey. Don't panic. God always has a way of providing everything we need at just the right time.

One of the best ways to experience God's provision is to start going to church. God's people know how to wrap their arms around a young mother and help her. Find a church where they teach the Bible and start attending regularly. As you get to know people, ask them to help you provide for your baby.

You have made it halfway through this book. Way to go! I am so proud of you for continuing your pregnancy journey with the Lord. Keep up the good work!

## EVENING PRAYER

Heavenly Father, it's an incredible thought that you have counted my baby's hairs; hair that will one day need to be combed, maybe even braided. If you have planned out my baby's hair, then surely you will help me prepare for and provide for this baby. Help my heart and mind to be ready to receive this baby. Help my home and my life to be ready to receive my child. When this precious person is finally placed into my arms, I pray that I will have everything I need. Please provide all the diapers, baby wipes, and clothes that I will need. I also need a crib and a baby stroller. I know that there are probably other things that I can't think of right now. Thank you, Lord, for providing everything I will need. I trust you! In Jesus' name, Amen.

# MORNING: DAY 11

## *YOUR BABY...*

## WILL BE MIGHTY

Praise the LORD. Blessed are those who fear the LORD, who find great delight in his commands. Their children will be mighty in the land; the generation of the upright will be blessed.
Psalm 112:1-2

God is able to do immeasurably more than all you can ask or imagine in and through your child (Eph 3:20). We don't dream big enough for our kids sometimes. The goal is not for them to be wealthy or successful. As you raise your child to know and love the Lord, God can do something so much bigger. God can make your child mighty!

As you live your life to please the Lord, God blesses you by blessing your child. God knows how much we love our children. He knows that this is one of the most wonderful things that He could ever do for us.

God can make your child "mighty in the land" one day. One day, people will look at your son or daughter and say, "Wow – there goes a great leader." Maybe they will say, "Who raised that incredible young man?" Your son or daughter could become a famous scientist or decorated military hero. God might even use your child to one day become a missionary or famous musician. God knows just how to make your child "mighty in the land."

Today, choose to do two things that you know will please the Lord. Maybe God has been gently encouraging you to do something that you have been avoiding. Maybe He wants you to forgive somebody or make a relationship right. Is there somebody in your life that you can reach out to for help? Obey the Lord not for your benefit, but so that you can save up blessings for your child. You can't make your child "mighty", but God can!

## EVENING PRAYER

Heavenly Father, it is an amazing thought that this child inside my womb could one day grow up to do amazing things. My child could someday comfort someone in need. My child could discover a cure for a terrible disease. My child could summon the courage to accomplish something great when everybody else is scared. My child could inspire the masses with poetry and effective leadership. Help my child to be mighty in the land!

Help me to be brave during this time of pregnancy. Help me to set an example for my child to follow. I want my child to see in my example what it looks like to make the right choices. Help me right now, this very minute, to be the mother this child needs. Help me to raise this baby to know you and to love you.

I'm so thankful that I do not have to do this alone, but that you are with me. Thank you for being with me every moment of every day. In Jesus' name, Amen.

# MORNING: DAY 12

## *YOUR BABY...*

## IS PART OF GOD'S STORY

Your eyes saw my unformed body; all the days ordained for me were written in your book before one of them came to be.
Psalm 139:16

God is writing a beautiful story! Did you know that you are an important part of God's story? God loves you and knows all about your life. Before you were even born, God saw your unformed body and knew everything about your future. Your pregnancy has not caught God by surprise. He has always known this wonderfully challenging season was coming for you. You might be shocked, but God is not.

Your baby is also an important part of God's story. Before your child is even born, God will know everything about the days of his or her life. God's story includes your precious unborn baby. We don't know anything about this story, but God knows everything.

Don't you want to know how your baby will be part of God's amazing story? Aren't you excited to see all the ways that the Lord will use your child? Not only do you get to watch this story unfold, but you get to be part of it. God wants you to raise your child to do all the things that He's already written about in His book. God wants you to teach your child how to walk and talk so that they can do everything He calls them to do. Somebody has to potty-train your baby and one day teach them how to ride a bike and drive a car.

Before you start your day, ask God for the strength to do the things that have to be done. Remember, you are an important part of God's story. God has great things in store for you and your baby. Each day is important. Remember, you don't have to do things in your own strength. Let God help you! Before you go to sleep tonight – don't forget your evening prayer!

## EVENING PRAYER

Heavenly Father, my life is part of your story and now this baby is a part of your story. As I think about the story of my life and the kind of story I would like for my baby, I know I need your help. I want my baby to feel loved, valued, special, and important. When I read your words in Psalm 139:16, it makes me feel amazed that you would want to include me in your story, that my life matters to you. If my story matters to you, then so does my baby's story. I pray for the story that my baby will live out. I pray that the story will be wonderful and that my baby will know of your love. May my child's story be filled with wonder and joy. Give my child a beautiful and happy life. In Jesus' name, Amen.

# MORNING: DAY 13

## *YOUR BABY...*

## NEEDS TO MEET JESUS

People were also bringing babies to Jesus
for him to place his hands on them.
Luke 18:15

You get to be the person that introduces your baby to all the special people in your life. You get to introduce your baby to your mom or dad. Won't it be wonderful to introduce your best friend to your baby? Do you have a sister or a brother that will be waiting in the hospital lobby to meet your baby? There is somebody even more important than these people in your life.

The most important person that you could ever introduce your child to is Jesus. Jesus wants to meet your child! One day your baby will be old enough for you to tell him or her about Jesus. You can read your child stories from a picture Bible and practice memory verses together. Your child will look to you for everything in life. If you introduce your child to Jesus, they will want to know all about Him. Your child needs to hear from you that Jesus loves them. You need to be the one that tells your child all about what Jesus did for them on the cross; that Jesus died so that they could be forgiven of their sins. One day you will get to tell your child about all the things that Jesus has done for you in your life. You can even tell your child how Jesus helped you through each day of your pregnancy. You get to be the one that teaches your child how to pray.

In order for you to introduce your child to Jesus, you need to make sure that you know Him. Do you know Jesus? When is the last time you read your Bible? Open the pages of the Bible and ask the Lord to reveal Himself to you. If you don't have a Bible, ask your local church or pregnancy center. They would be happy to give you a free one. Spend a few moments reading the New Testament. God will bless you as you get to know Jesus.

Mom – you have such an important job! If you introduce your child to Jesus, you will have accomplished the most important thing that a mother can do.

## EVENING PRAYER

Heavenly Father, so many people have disappointed me, but I am trusting that you will never disappoint me. Help me to understand that you love me and will never leave me. Help me to teach my baby that, although other people come and go, you will always be there. I pray that my baby would know you and want to be like you. Help my child to love you. I pray that my baby would always know your love. In Jesus' name, Amen.

# MORNING: DAY 14

## *Your Baby...*

## IS YOUR FAMILY

God sets the lonely in families.
Psalm 68:6

Do you have a family? You may be blessed with a wonderful family full of people who love and care for you. You might have the kind of parents who are always there for you when you need them. Sadly, not everybody has a great family. Maybe that describes you. This very minute you might not have anybody to turn to for love and support. Everybody needs a family. Are you ready for some great news? God is giving you a new family member!

God loves you so much that He is giving you a family member who will love you more than you could ever imagine. Your baby is now your family. You now have a blood relative that is always going to love you just the way you are.

God sets the lonely in families. God is giving you a best friend who will love you the rest of your life. God is giving you a child that will fill your life with joy and delight. One day your child will call and text you on the phone. You are going to experience every Christmas together. Imagine enjoying a steaming cup of hot chocolate around a warm fire on Christmas Eve. Imagine carving a perfectly cooked turkey on Thanksgiving Day or baking cookies together. You are going to make wonderful memories in your family.

It's hard to imagine right now, but one day your child will be old enough to take care of you. When you are old and grey, you will have a strong, capable adult who can care for your needs the way that you cared for them. God knows that everyone needs a family. You now have one. Get ready to enjoy the best of life with your new family member.

## EVENING PRAYER

Heavenly Father, I am facing so many emotions. I am excited one moment and scared the next over how my life is about to change. Protect me from negative people who will discourage me from choosing life for my baby. Help me to be strong and stand up for my baby. My baby is my family now. You are the One who makes families. Help my new family to be strong and happy. Surround me with people who will encourage me. Send a special friend into my life to support me as I transition into motherhood. In Jesus' name, Amen.

## MORNING: DAY 15

*YOUR BABY...*

# CAN GIVE YOU GRANDCHILDREN

May you live to see your children's children...
Psalm 128:6

The only thing more wonderful than having children is having grandchildren. I know it's hard to imagine during the early stages of your pregnancy, but the day is coming when your child will get married and very likely have a child of their own. One of the greatest blessings of God is living long enough to see "your children's children." Maybe you will be "Nana" or "Mimi." Can you imagine experiencing all the joy of little ones while having only a fraction of the responsibility?

Not only does God see your baby's baby, but He knows the multitude that will come from your child. From the child in your womb God can bring about a multitude of people. Your child may one day have grandchildren and great-grandchildren of their own. Isn't this amazing? Think about this for a moment. From the child in your womb, God knows about every schoolteacher, policeman, fireman, doctor, lawyer, counselor, and pastor that He will bring into the world. He knows about every contribution that all of them will make to society. Your baby is more important to God than you could ever imagine! Bringing your baby into the world might be the most important accomplishment that you will ever have.

Given how important the job of motherhood is, it's so important that you take care of yourself during your pregnancy. Are you getting plenty of rest? Are you eating healthy and drinking plenty of water? It's also important to exercise. Have you been going to all of your doctor visits? Be sure not to miss these important visits. Take care of yourself, because no one else can do the job of bringing your baby into the world!

## EVENING PRAYER

Heavenly Father, help me to leave a legacy through my child and one day through my grandchildren. Help me to leave a legacy of strength. Right now, I need strength to say "yes" to the right things and "no" to the wrong things. Help me to be strong through all the challenges of pregnancy and motherhood. I also want to leave a legacy of love. I want my baby to grow up knowing that they are loved and special. Help me to teach my baby what true love looks like. Help me to make a big impact on the world through raising my child. In Jesus' name, Amen.

# MORNING: DAY 16

## *YOUR BABY...*

## HAS A GOOD SHEPHERD

The LORD is my shepherd, I lack nothing.
He makes me lie down in green pastures,
he leads me beside quiet waters, he refreshes my soul. He guides me along the right paths for his name's sake. Even though I walk through the darkest valley, I will fear no evil, for you are with me; your rod and your staff they comfort me. You prepare a table before me in the presence of my enemies. You anoint my head with oil;
my cup overflows. Surely your goodness and love will follow me all the days of my life, and I will dwell in the house of the LORD forever.
Psalm 23

We live in a world filled with hardship and pain. Have you ever thought to yourself, "How could I bring a child into this messed-up world?" If you have, you are not alone.

Our world is filled with problems. But don't let the problems of this world keep you from the wonder and beauty of bringing a precious baby into the world. Here is why. There is a power mightier than the biggest problems of this world. There is a light that can brighten the deepest darkness. There is a God who is Lord over all the chaos. No matter how difficult things are for your child, they will have a Good Shepherd to guide them through life.

As your child follows the Lord, He will care for all their physical needs. God is a wonderful provider; He will lead your child into the best pastures in life. Knowing your child's weaknesses and frailties, God will lead them to gentle waters.

As the perfect Shepherd, God also knows how to care for your child's spiritual needs. No doctor, life-coach, mentor, or pastor can care for your child's spiritual needs in the ways that God can. God knows how to knit every broken piece of our soul back together.

The Good Shepherd will also be faithful to guide your child through all the confusing seasons of life. God is the perfect guide through all the storms of life. Even when your child goes through valleys in life, they will not need to fear. God is armed with the perfect arsenal to comfort your child.

The Good Shepherd can also bless your child with abundant joy even through the most challenging times in life. Your child never has to be alone in life.

The Good Shepherd promises to pursue His flock throughout their entire life. Your child will never be alone. Psalm 23 ends with a wonderful promise. When we die having lived our life following the Good Shepherd, we enjoy the privilege of dwelling "in the house of the Lord forever."

Did you know that God wants to be your Good Shepherd as well? As you place your faith and trust in Jesus for the forgiveness of your sin, you can experience the joys of having a Good Shepherd care for you. If you have not already done so, take a moment and commit yourself to following Jesus as your Lord and Savior! You don't have to be alone through this pregnancy journey. Turn to the Good Shepherd and trust Him to care for all your physical and spiritual needs.

## EVENING PRAYER

Heavenly Father, what a comfort it is to know that I do not have to walk through this life alone. You are always with me. Please provide for me during this challenging season of life. You know all the physical, emotional and spiritual needs that I have. Guide me, protect me, and comfort me. Please give me an overflowing cup of joy today. I trust you to care for me in every good way. What a comfort it is to know that you will always be with my baby. You will take perfect care of my baby. I pray that your goodness would be poured out lavishly on my baby. May you pursue my child with your love their entire life. May all the days of my child's life be filled with praises for your name! In Jesus' name, Amen.

# MORNING: DAY 17

## *Your Baby...*

## HAS A FUTURE

"For I know the plans I have for you," declares the LORD, "plans to prosper you and not to harm you, plans to give you hope and a future."
Jeremiah 29:11

I believe God has amazing plans for your baby! When you and I make plans, things don't always go the way that we want. Our inability to follow through, combined with the unpredictable nature of our world, means that our plans sometimes fail. Sometimes our plans fail because they are selfish or because they are not realistic.

In contrast, God's plans are always perfect. There is not one flaw in God's plan for your baby! God's plan for your baby does not include harm. Don't let anybody tell you that hurting your baby is the right thing. God would never make a plan that includes harming your baby. God has plans to prosper your baby. God wants your baby to grow up to do incredible things. God wants to give your baby hope and a future. I know that it seems impossible right now to provide a great future for your baby. Rest assured, you are not alone. God has a plan for your baby's future.

God also has a powerful ability to follow through and make His plan happen. What a joy it will be to sit back and watch God carry out His perfect plan for your baby! Not only do you get to observe God at work in your child's life, but you will get to actively participate in it. You are not alone as you raise your child. God wants to come alongside you so that His perfect plan for your baby is completed.

Did you know that God has plans for you as well? Even before you were born, God had plans to prosper you; plans to give you hope and a future. Commit yourself to the Lord this day. Tell God that you are ready to do life His way. Tell God that you want to experience the plan that He made for you a long time ago. It's never too late to say "yes" to God. It's never too late to obey the Lord. God wants to give you hope and a future! Be encouraged today!

## EVENING PRAYER

Heavenly father, what a joy I feel when I hear that you are with me – when I hear that you have a plan for my life. I find comfort knowing I'm not alone. I need you to be with me each and every day. Right now, I know that your plan involves having this baby. Thank you that you have a wonderful future for me and this baby. I don't know who my baby will grow up to be, but you do. I know that you have a great plan for my child. I pray that you would do incredible things through my baby's life. Help me to awake tomorrow morning excited about the plans you have for me! In Jesus' name, Amen.

# MORNING: DAY 18

## *YOUR BABY...*

## WILL BLESS YOU

Her children arise and call her blessed…
Proverbs 31:28

One day, your child will grow old enough to understand what a great mother you are. One day, he or she will understand just how frightened and overwhelmed you were to be pregnant. One day, they will understand the sacrifices you made to bring them into the world. One day, they will comprehend the strength it took for you to do the right thing. One day, your child will rise and call you "blessed."

You may not feel like a great mom yet, but you are. Right now, you are caring for your baby in a way that nobody else can. Nobody else can provide a womb for your baby to grow and mature in. Nobody else can make sure that your child receives the nourishment and protection that they need. Only you can do this for your baby. You are already being a great mother. One day, your child will thank you for it. You might have to wait a long time, but the day is coming when your child realizes what you did for them.

Even more important than their gratitude will be when they choose to follow your courageous example. One day, when they are tempted to do the wrong thing, they will remember how hard you worked to do the right thing in bringing them into the world. The strength of your example will be a blessing to them for many years to come. Your obedience in bringing your baby into the world might impact generations!

Today, I want to encourage you to go back to church this Sunday. I know it sounds hard to do, but your baby needs you to be in a safe, loving environment where you can learn more about the Lord. Your baby needs you to grow strong in the Lord during this pregnancy.

## EVENING PRAYER

Heavenly Father, give me the strength to raise this baby. Help me to remember that one day this baby will grow into a loving and caring adult. One day, this baby could grow up and be my best friend. Right now, it is hard to believe that my choice to raise my child could be an example of strength, but I pray that it will be. I pray that I would make many strong choices that will help my baby to grow into the incredible person you want them to be. I pray that when my child grows up, they will be proud of their mother. I also pray for the strength to find a church. I need a church that will love me and my baby. I need a church that will teach both of us about You and Your Word. In Jesus' name, Amen.

# MORNING: DAY 19

## *Your Baby...*

## TREASURED BY JESUS

Jesus said, "Let the little children come to me, and do not hinder them, for the kingdom of heaven belongs to such as these."
Matthew 19:14

Jesus wants all the children to come to Him! Jesus wants children from every country and every ethnicity to come to Him. There is not a single child that Jesus does not want to be around. In Matthew 19, people were bringing their children to Jesus. Some of the cranky adults around Jesus thought it was a nuisance, but Jesus loved it. He wanted to place His loving hands on them and bless them. Jesus told those cranky adults that "the kingdom of heaven belongs to such as these." If we want to know how to inherit salvation and heaven, then we need the simple, whole-hearted, faith of children. Children are ready to believe in Jesus. They are ready to follow Jesus and worship

Jesus. Every adult needs the constant reminders to be more like children.

Your baby is not a burden or a complication to your life. God wants to teach you so much through your child. Through raising your child, you will learn so much about the woman God has called you to be.

You are going to make it through this challenging season of pregancy. I know it probably seems like it will never end, but I promise you – it will. In fact, today you are closer to your delivery than you have ever been. When you finally have the joy of holding your baby for the first time, you will begin the beautiful journey of leading your child to Jesus. Jesus wants you to bring your child to Him. This is one of the great reasons to be involved in a local, Bible-believing Christian Church.

Your child needs you to bring them to church. Your child needs you to tell them Bible stories at night. Your child needs you to teach them how to pray to the Lord. Your child needs you to teach them about wrong and right. There is no better person to teach your child these lessons. Bringing your child to Jesus is the most important thing that you could ever do with your life.

When you get tired and weary, I want you to say the words of Jesus to yourself, "Let the little children come to me." When you are nauseous and scared about the future, repeat those beautiful words to yourself. Every time people tell you not to have your baby, repeat those wonderful words to yourself. Again and again, remind yourself that Jesus wants all the little children to come to Him!

## EVENING PRAYER

Heavenly Father, as I get to know you, I am amazed at how much you love babies, children, and mothers. When so many people around me tell me that children are a problem, help me to remember how you love and treasure them. I pray that you would fill my heart with a desire to teach my child about you. Please give my child a desire to learn all about you. I pray that my child would spend their entire life loving you and growing close to you.

# MORNING: DAY 20

## *YOUR BABY...*

## IS A BLESSING FROM THE LORD

Children are a heritage from the LORD,
offspring a reward from him.
Like arrows in the hands of a warrior
are children born in one's youth.
Blessed is the man whose quiver is full of them.
Psalm 127:3-5

You are blessed! Were you shocked to find out you were pregnant? Were you stressed out and overwhelmed? I bet you were also a little scared at the road ahead of you. These are normal emotions when it comes to unplanned pregnancies. You can be all those things and blessed at the same time. It may not feel like it in this moment, but you are blessed! You don't have to feel blessed to be blessed. Children are a blessing from the Lord!

In Psalm 127, God compares children to a

reward! You have basically won the lottery of God's blessing! No amount of money or worldly possessions could be as wonderful as a baby made in the image of God, unlike the things of this world that will tarnish and fade with time. Your baby will grow big and strong with time. Your baby has a soul that can experience the rest of all eternity with the Lord.

Psalm 127 also says that your child is like an arrow in the hand of a warrior. No warrior could go to battle without his arrows. Arrows represent strength and victory. One day, God may use your child to do great things.

Babies are not complications in your life. They are not a nuisance or a burden. Babies are blessings from the Lord. Don't run from God's blessing. Don't be afraid of God's blessing. Embrace the blessing by embracing your baby! Today, give thanks for God's blessings.

## EVENING PRAYER

Heavenly Father, thank you for this baby who will be a blessing to me in my life. When I feel overwhelmed and scared, help me to remember that this child is a blessing from you. Help me to embrace this wonderful blessing with all my heart. Throughout the rest of this pregnancy, help me to find comfort in your words. Help me to find joy in knowing that you have a plan for me and my child. Thank you for loving me and for loving my baby. Help me to raise this baby with all my heart and to experience all the joys that you have for my new family. I know that I can trust you to provide everything I need to be a great mother. Thank you for my baby! In Jesus' name, Amen.

# CLOSING THOUGHTS

## YOU MADE IT!

You made it! I am so proud of you for reading this entire book. Way to Go. God will bless you for caring enough about your baby to read this book. You have chosen to share your unforgettable pregnancy experience with the Lord. While you are finished reading this book, your pregnancy journey might be far from over. Whether you have 4 more months to go or 4 more weeks to go, keep doing what you have been doing. Keep reading the Bible and going to church. Keep praying to the Lord every day for strength. Keep making healthy choices for your baby. Stay connected with your local pregnancy center. There are so many ways that they can help you in the weeks and months to come. God is going to bless you for doing the right thing. We are so proud of you.

# RESOURCES FOR UNPLANNED PREGNANCIES

- Go to OptionLine.org to find a Pregnancy Resource Center. Or, call their confidential Hotline 800-712-4357 or Text "Helpline" to 313131.

- Go to MyChoiceNetwork.org to find a Pregnancy Resource Center.

- Call Care Net for help or to connect with a local pregnancy center: M-F 10am - 6pm EST 877-791-5475.

- Reach out to the nearest Bible-believing Christian Church for assistance.

## ENCOURAGING BIBLE VERSES

**Psalm 46:1** God is our refuge and strength, an ever-present help in trouble.

**Psalm 103:8** The Lord is compassionate and gracious, slow to anger, abounding in love.

**Isaiah 41:10** So do not fear, for I am with you; do not be dismayed, for I am your God. I will strengthen you and help you; I will uphold you with my righteous right hand.

**Romans 8:28** And we know that in all things God works for the good of those who love him, who have been called according to his purpose.

**Romans 15:13** May the God of hope fill you with all joy and peace as you trust in him, so that you may overflow with hope by the power of the Holy Spirit.

**Philippians 4:6-7** Do not be anxious about anything, but in every situation, by prayer and petition, with thanksgiving, present your requests to God. And the peace of God, which transcends all understanding, will guard your hearts and your minds in Christ Jesus.

**Philippians 4:13** I can do all this through him who gives me strength.

**I John 1:9** If we confess our sins, he is faithful and just and will forgive us our sins and purify us from all unrighteousness.

# ENDORSEMENTS

"Every devotional is written through the lens of scripture and therefore has the power to transform lives by the working of the Holy Spirit. Each evening prayer will bring comfort and peace and confidence that, 'God's got this, so I can sleep peacefully tonight!' This devotional is really like a love letter from God to Moms."

Libby Bogged
Client Advocate, Thrive Women's Center
Dallas, TX

"This charming little book is easy to read and encourages expectant mothers to not only ponder the amazing plans that God has set forth for their little one; but to also understand her very important role in that plan. I believe this book would make an excellent resource for Pregnancy Centers and their clients."

Eve Roberts
CEO, Wise Choices P.R.C.
Decatur, TX

"It's as if God wrote a prophetic vision of the value of an unborn person and bound it in this book!"

Dean Polk
Board Chair, Huntsville Pregnancy Resource Center
Huntsville, AL

"A must read for expecting mothers! God's truth in a practical, straightforward manner."

Steve Perkins
Board Member, Wise Choices P.R.C.
Decatur, TX

"Each day is filled with gems of hope!"

Roberta Cheek
Executive Director, CareNet P.R.C. of Santa Fe
Santa Fe, NM

## ABOUT THE AUTHORS

Kevin and Stephanie are joyfully married and are blessed with four children. Stephanie has a love for art, beauty, and homeschooling her children. Kevin loves music, writing books, rock climbing, and preaching God's Word. Raising their children is one of their greatest joys in life.

## Connect with Kevin and Stephanie

We would love to hear how the Lord used this book to help you or someone you love make a life-affirming choice.

Are you interested in donating copies of *Your Baby…* to your local pregnancy center? We would love to discuss ways of doing that.

Here is how you can connect with us…

Website: www.kevinjmoore.me

Email: authorkevinjmoore@gmail.com

Facebook: Facebook.com/authorkevinmoore

Made in the USA
Coppell, TX
05 October 2023

22462390R00049